Dr. K's Sure-Fire INSTANT Weight-Loss SECRETS

Personal Growth Books
Forthcoming from KoPubCo

Who Moved My Rich Dad?

The One-Minute Employee

The Automatic Pauper

The Seven Hobbits of
Highly Successful Paladins

Cracking the Millionaire Codpiece

What Color Is Your Stool?

Dr. K's Sure-Fire INSTANT Weight-Loss SECRETS

by
"Dr. K"

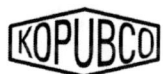

First Printing, August 2009

Copyright © 2009 by The Triplanetary Corporation

ISBN 10 0-9777649-6-6
ISBN 13 978-0-9777649-6-9

Published by arrangement with the author.

All rights reserved. No part of this book may be reproduced, emitted, or transmitted in any form by any means—electronic or mechanical, including photocopying, recording, or by any information storage and retrieval system—without permission in writing from the publisher.

KoPubCo—publishing division of
The Triplanetary Corporation
5942 Edinger Ave., Ste. 113-164
Huntington Beach, California 92649
www.kopubco.com

KOPUBCO and the KoPubCo colophons are trademarks of the Triplanetary Corporation.

Printed by Lightning Source, Inc.

Cover designed by Black Dawn Graphics

This book is dedicated to my wife,
who could use a good laugh

This Page Intentionally Left Blank

[no... wait... now it's not... *dammit!*]

Table of Contents

Preface 13

Chapter 1: How to Lose Weight 15

Chapter 2: The Secret of Strength 19

Chapter 3: Dealing With Setbacks 23

Chapter 4: How to Handle Sabotage 27

Chapter 5: Finding Balance in Your Life 31

Chapter 6: You Can Find the Power to Win! 35

Chapter 7: The Secret to Success in Work 39

Chapter 8: The Secret to Success at Sex 43

Chapter 9: The Secret to Success at Life 47

Chapter 10: How to Find More Time and Energy 51

Chapter 11: The Secret to Long Life 55

Chapter 12: How Olympic Athletes Do It 59

Chapter 13: Why Super-Models Look So Hot 63

Chapter 14: When You Feel the Urge to Cheat 67

Chapter 15: How to Lose Those Thighs 71

Chapter 16: How to Look Sexy at Any Age 75

Chapter 17: The Way to Banish Love Handles 79

Chapter 18: Arms the Size of Ham Hocks? 83

Chapter 19: Finding Your Forgotten Abs 87

Chapter 20: The Final Secret 91

Afterword 95

Index 97

Dr. K's Sure-Fire INSTANT Weight-Loss SECRETS

Disclaimer

Before embarking on any diet or exercise regimen (or regime or regiment, for that matter), check with your doctor. In fact, if you are planning to follow the directions of a book that's labeled "humor" on its spine, maybe you should also check with your psychiatrist. Exercising and changing your eating patterns both involve significant risk of injury or death. Of course, doing nothing differently in your life can lead to bloating, muscular degeneration, BO, explosive flatulence, and death. Really, anything we do eventually leads to death, right, so why even try? As Luke Rhinehart said in *The Dice Man*, "Life is islands of ecstasy in an ocean of ennui, and after the age of thirty land is seldom seen." Geez, what was wrong with that guy? Lighten up. That's what *est* will do to you.

Please use your locker for all valuables and do not leave the gym for any reason. This is not a contract, no warranties are implied or should be inferred, and no bailment is created. All articles excluded shall be deemed included. Author completely denies everything. He's not even a professionally trained writer. He just threw this together during a bender and can't figure out how it got typeset and published. He thinks a Muse did it, but he may have just been listening to the original cast album of *Xanadu on Broadway*. And no, he's not gay, he just likes a good show tune now and then. Nothing gay about that. *Nothing at all!*

Watch the free book-on-video featuring "Dr. K" at www.kopubco.com/video/secrets.html

Preface

Thousands of books have been written about weight loss. Some of them are diet books—low-fat diets, low-carb diets, all-meat diets, hummingbird-tongue diets, pulverized-coprolite diets. Other weight-loss books strive to change your lifestyle, such as urging you to take up yoga, or live like Uzbeks, or emulate wine-swilling, pasta-scarfing Mediterraneans.

Screw that. My system is much simpler. *Simple, but not easy,* you may be asking yourself? *Nah*—easy, too. BTW, do you talk to yourself a lot? Better get that checked.

In the following pages, you will find the absolute, incontrovertible secrets of weight loss that will take you from fat to fabulous, from weak to wonderful, and from slothful to sexy. Follow them scrupulously, and you will be rewarded far beyond your wildest dreams of slenderness.

What have you got to lose, but fat itself?

— *Dr. K*

"Dr. K"

Chapter One
How to Lose Weight

This is the first and toughest question one asks oneself, except perhaps for "Where am I, why am I naked, and how did my car end up in the liquor aisle?" You can read an entire diet and exercise book and only in the very last chapter will you come to The Secret at which the author has only vaguely hinted. I'm not going to mess around with your head that way. You're in a hurry to lose weight and lead a better life, so turn the page and read Dr. K's prescription for Instant, Sure-Fire Weight Loss!

"Dr. K"

EAT LESS!

Dr. K's Sure-Fire Instant Weight-Loss Secrets

EXERCISE MORE!

"Dr. K"

Chapter Two
The Secret of Strength

Wasn't that easy? Weight loss is simple math: burn more calories than you eat. You can accomplish this either by eating less (fewer calories in) or exercising more (more calories burnt). Doing *both* multiplies the effect. Building up your strength ranks right behind weight loss as one of the most important aspects of feeling better and looking younger. It also helps to hang around with older, flabbier people. People ask if they should exercise using steroids. I say, whatever helps. I usually put a Pat Benatar album on my steroid, crank it up, and just rock out while I exercise. Some people use their iPod, but I avoid them because I was so freaked out by that creepy old movie *Invasion of the Body Snatchers*. How do you burn fat and build muscle? Read on!

"Dr. K"

EAT LESS!

Dr. K's Sure-Fire Instant Weight-Loss Secrets

EXERCISE MORE!

"Dr. K"

Chapter Three
DEALING WITH SETBACKS

In our quest for health, we all sometimes take two steps forward and one step back. If you find that you are consistently taking *one* step forward and *two* steps back, for God's sake turn around—you may not be making any progress, but you'll *think* you are, and that's all you can ask from most weight-loss programs. But this isn't just *any* run-of-the-treadmill program. This is the one that *works*, guaranteed!* So how do you handle those times when all your efforts don't seem to be enough and your scale shows that you've hit that notorious plateau?

---

* Guarantee void wherever warranties are legally enforceable.

"Dr. K"

EAT LESS!

Dr. K's Sure-Fire Instant Weight-Loss Secrets

EXERCISE MORE!

"Dr. K"

Chapter Four
HOW TO HANDLE SABOTAGE FROM FRIENDS & FAMILY

Family. Can't live with 'em, can't risk being profiled by Keith Morrison on a special episode of *Dateline*. So what do you do when your conniving husband brings home a cake in a misguided effort to cheer you up? Forget the fact that you *asked* him to bring home cake—he should know better than to listen to *you* (he never does when you tell him anything else). How do you tell your kids that eating a sack of Bugles in front of you is not just unhelpful, but is the fast-track to a visit from Child Protective Services? The best solution is to take a deep breath, calmly tell your coworkers that Dollar Margarita Night is a bad idea, and do the following...

"Dr. K"

EAT LESS!

Dr. K's Sure-Fire Instant Weight-Loss Secrets

EXERCISE MORE!

"Dr. K"

Chapter Five

FINDING BALANCE IN YOUR LIFE

Work. Sleep. Family. Friends. You. Is that how you structure your life? Or is it Work. Sleep. Work. Sleep. Work. Sleep. Work. Sleep. Work. Sleep. Work. Sleep. Work. Sleep. Work. Sleep. Work. Sleep. Work. Sleep. Work. Myocardial Infarction? A balanced life means more than a banana Daiquiri in one hand and a banana split in the other. It means taking a good long look at what is most important to you, deciding what portion of each day should be devoted to what, then chucking it all because you had been assured that there would be no math. Balancing your life is much simpler; you only need to count to two!

"Dr. K"

1.
EAT
LESS!

2.
EXERCISE MORE!

"Dr. K"

Chapter Six
YOU CAN FIND THE POWER TO WIN!

Winning is not the main thing. It's not even the *only* thing. Winning is *the* thing. James Arness was *The Thing*. Therefore, Winning is James Arness. (By logical extension, James Arness is also Michael Chiklis.) Winning is something you should be doing every day, like showering or sex (see chapter 8). Or sex while showering. Sorry, my mind wandered for a second there. The point is, your mind should be constantly focused on *winning*. A weak, flabby body leads to a weak, flabby mind that will never win the marathon of life and will look simultaneously disgusting and hilarious trying to run it. The road to winning begins with two small steps:

"Dr. K"

EAT LESS!

Dr. K's Sure-Fire Instant Weight-Loss Secrets

EXERCISE MORE!

"Dr. K"

Dr. K's Sure-Fire Instant Weight-Loss Secrets

Chapter Seven
THE SECRET TO SUCCESS AT WORK

How many overweight weaklings are truly successful at work? I mean, besides your Congressman and every website developer you've ever met? Studies have shown that slim, fit employees earn more than their roly-poly counterparts. And they save more, too, since they don't have to budget for donuts, Dockers with the "relaxed fit," or second seats on airplanes. Want to get through the work day without being elbowed awake by a co-worker? How about being able to punch your cellphone keys without using a pencil eraser? Any desire to avoid reading a paragraph in the company's disaster plan solely devoted to evacuating *you*? Then do this:

"Dr. K"

EAT LESS!

Dr. K's Sure-Fire Instant Weight-Loss Secrets

EXERCISE MORE!

"Dr. K"

Chapter Eight

THE SECRET TO SUCCESS AT SEX

Health plays an important role in sexual satisfaction. If you are out of shape and overweight, you decrease your chances of finding a mate or—if you do find one—of surviving the episode. You don't want to make love on the seashore only to have concerned beachgoers roll you into the ocean so you can rejoin your migrating pod. (Again, enough about pods.) Why is it that all the slender, smoothly muscled people get all the men/women/trannies they want? *Because they look good. Duh!* But why is thin nearly always in? Because we evolved on the African Savannah to be strong, fast, and capable of hiding behind blades of grass. And that image is burned into our collective sexual unconscious the same way Hayden Panettiere and Jimmy Fallon are.

"Dr. K"

EAT LESS!

Dr. K's Sure-Fire Instant Weight-Loss Secrets

EXERCISE MORE!

"Dr. K"

Chapter Nine
THE SECRET TO SUCCESS AT LIFE

Some will say that the secret to success at life is to achieve some kind of immortality. Some achieve immortality through their works. Some achieve it through a child. Filmmaker Woody Allen quipped that he wanted to achieve immortality by not dying. Come to think of it, Woody achieved it through Mia Farrow's child. However you achieve immortality, you don't want attached to it the prefix "World's Fattest..." Success at life is achieved through *living*, and the best way to keep living is through *health*. Success at living is not defined as successfully waking up between each bout of apnea or having enough plaque pulled out of your arteries to ice a sheet cake. So...

"Dr. K"

EAT LESS!

Dr. K's Sure-Fire Instant Weight-Loss Secrets

EXERCISE MORE!

"Dr. K"

Chapter Ten
How to Find More Time and Energy

Okay, Einstein, I know mass can't be created or destroyed—it can only be converted into energy and back again. The whole point of this book is to explain how *you* can convert that mass around your thighs into energy and radiate it away from you. Sure, you'll be increasing entropy, but the whole universe is flying apart due to Dark Energy (which is *not* the new Gatorade drink), so don't worry. And I know time is relative: you can't get any more hours in a day, but they *can* feel absolutely interminable when spent on a Stairclimber. When you burn fat, guess what? That burnt fat is *energy*, which boosts your metabolism like a grease fire at KFC.

"Dr. K"

EAT LESS!

Dr. K's Sure-Fire Instant Weight-Loss Secrets

EXERCISE MORE!

"Dr. K"

Chapter Eleven
THE SECRET TO LONG LIFE

Quality of life is ultimately just as important as *quantity* of life. It's the same for food: what good is a sack of six White Castle burgers when they're *White Castle burgers?* More of something that's bad is not good (leave sex out of this) (*see Chapter 8*). So a *long* life also needs to be a *good* life. And—amazingly enough—a good, healthy life tends to promote a long life. People who live fast and die young rarely leave a good-looking corpse, *viz.* John Belushi, Chris Farley, and The Notorious B.I.G. On the other hand, Jack LaLanne is in his nineties and follows the Dr. K plan to the letter:

"Dr. K"

EAT LESS!

EXERCISE MORE!

"Dr. K"

Chapter Twelve
How Olympic Athletes Do It

Now some of you may be thinking that eating less and exercising more is too simplistic. After all, exercising can increase your body's need for fuel, and once you've burned off that fat like a Japanese whaler renders a ton of blubber, eating less may actually leave you with too few calories to supply your new metabolism with everything it needs to keep your body going. So eat *more*. Sheesh, what am I, your mother? Don't get me started on my mother, walking in while I'm... *meditating* on my Cheryl Ladd poster and saying "As long as you're not doing anything, take out the garbage." I'll bet Michael Phelps doesn't have time to take out the garbage when he's eating 12,000 calories a day...

"Dr. K"

EAT
MORE

Dr. K's Sure-Fire Instant Weight-Loss Secrets

BUT EXERCISE INSANELY

"Dr. K"

Chapter Thirteen
Why Supermodels Look So Hot

Good Lord, do I even have to explain this?

"Dr. K"

EAT LESS!

Dr. K's Sure-Fire Instant Weight-Loss Secrets

EXERCISE MORE!

"Dr. K"

Chapter Fourteen
WHEN YOU FEEL THE URGE TO CHEAT

After thirteen chapters of intense, step-by-step instruction, I should think you won't be prone to backslide, since your backside should be so small by now that you won't be sliding off of anything. But just in case you decide to eat *more* and exercise *less*, keep this in mind: even Dorothy Lamour would look bad in a muu-muu and you can't wear a slinky, sexy sarong if your ass is as wide as Mauna Loa. Feeling guilty? Good! I'm a great proponent of guilt. A guilty conscience is proof that you know the difference between right and wrong, so embrace your guilt and listen to it. When you feel the urge to cheat, just keep this chapter bookmarked and turn to it for its simple words of wisdom:

"Dr. K"

EAT LESS!

EXERCISE MORE!

"Dr. K"

Chapter Fifteen
How to Lose Those Thighs

The notion of spot-reducing has been proven to be about as effective as trying to empty out the center of a gravy boat: the gravy surrounding it slurps in to foil your efforts. Those thighs aren't going to shrink down if the rest of your body looks like a titanic matzoh ball. You could do ten thousand leg-presses and if it isn't accompanied by some aerobic, fat-burning exercise, those mighty thigh muscles will just push the everything outward and you'll look like Eddie Murphy in a fat suit. The only way to lose fat in one part of you is to lose fat *everywhere*. Happily, there are only two things you have to do to lose that fat:

"Dr. K"

EAT LESS!

Dr. K's Sure-Fire Instant Weight-Loss Secrets

EXERCISE MORE!

"Dr. K"

Chapter Sixteen
How to Look Sexy at Any Age

Some people are sexy no matter what their age, like Goldie Hawn, Sean Connery, Christie Brinkley, Raquel Welch, Richard Gere, Harrison Ford, and Charo. Some people aren't: Rosie O'Donnell, Michael Moore, Carnie Wilson, Bruce Vilanch. Some started out sexy and then something went horribly wrong: Marlon Brando, Elvis Presley, Kirstie Alley, ALF. What is the dividing line? Overweight. Out of shape. Falling in love with the cannoli. The key to looking sexy at any age is to stay trim and stay alive. How many obese people over seventy do you know? That's because they're *dead*. Dead isn't sexy. Want to know how the longest-living stars stay sexy? Read on!

"Dr. K"

EAT LESS!

EXERCISE MORE!

"Dr. K"

Chapter Seventeen
THE WAY TO BANISH LOVE HANDLES

Men suffer from this malady more than women, although the dreaded Muffin Top is the distaff equivalent of the Love Handle. If you don't believe there's any reason your lover should be able to carry you like a suitcase, then maybe you should think about ditching the spare tire. Remember what I said about spot reducing, though. The only way to lose that equatorial bulge encircling Planet You is to lose *all* the fat. Get on that Exercycle and spin as if the Frito Bandito were hot on your tail (if you actually *eat* Fritos, he's already taken up residence).

"Dr. K"

EAT LESS!

Dr. K's Sure-Fire Instant Weight-Loss Secrets

EXERCISE MORE!

"Dr. K"

Dr. K's Sure-Fire Instant Weight-Loss Secrets

Chapter Eighteen
ARMS THE SIZE OF HAM HOCKS?

This may also be a guy problem, but nothing is worse on a woman than upper arms as thick and bulging as Popeye's. There's no way to shrink those caveman clubs other than to schlep over to the gym and *work your ass off* (which also has the added benefit of *working your ass off*). If you want forever to banish those baobab tree trunks you call arms, get out on the dance floor and aerobicize those pendulous sacks of schmaltz until they sizzle and sear away. So trust the good Dr. K: once you burn away the fat, whatever remains—no matter how unfamiliar it looks—is muscle. If you want to be more Hippolyta than hippo, take these two simple actions:

"Dr. K"

EAT LESS!

EXERCISE MORE!

"Dr. K"

Chapter Nineteen

THE SECRET TO FINDING YOUR FORGOTTEN ABS

You probably have a lovely set of abdominal muscles. They're simply hidden beneath a layer of... let's call it adipose tissue. You can do a thousand crunches a day or spend a fortune on the latest Abdominizerator Rocket Roller Tummy Genie™ and think you're going to have a killer six-pack, but unless you lose the mutton around your midriff, no one's going to see those chiseled mounds through the blanket of blubber enveloping them. You need to do aerobic, fat-burning workouts, too, in addition to the muscle-building exercises. Otherwise, all that muscle you build will be used solely for supporting your weight against the pull of gravity—not just Earth's, but your own!

"Dr. K"

EAT LESS!

Dr. K's Sure-Fire Instant Weight-Loss Secrets

EXERCISE MORE!

"Dr. K"

Chapter Twenty

THE FINAL SECRET TO AVOIDING SLEEP APNEA, DIABETES, GALLSTONES, HYPERTENSION, HEART DISEASE, EARLY DEATH, AND CANKLES

By now, it should be obvious...

"Dr. K"

EAT LESS!

EXERCISE MORE!

"Dr. K"

Dr. K's Sure-Fire Instant Weight-Loss Secrets

AFTERWORD

So there you have it: Dr. K's Sure-Fire Instant Weight-Loss Secrets. If you follow them, you will lose weight and be stronger than you ever imagined. Simple? Astonishingly, *yes!*

I know it seems difficult to believe, but all modern science and dozens of broad-based studies—double-blind, triple-blind, and even one totally blind and partially deaf—indicate that these previously undisclosed secrets are the *key* to weight loss and greater strength, stamina, and overall robust health.

I know this is news to you. No one has ever put into one book *all* the secrets of weight loss along with a step-by-step plan customized for *you*. Trust Dr. K*, follow the plan in this book religiously, and see results virtually overnight. Maybe overmonth, but, anyway, science is on your side!

Good luck, good health, good riddance.

---

* Dr. K is not a medical doctor, but *is* working on his Ph.D. in medieval literature.

"Dr. K"

This edition of *Dr. K's Sure-Fire Instant Weight-Loss Secrets* is set in Century Schoolbook type, a very pleasant and readable font, at 12 points on 14 point leading. Titles are in Baskerville Old Face. Typesetting, layout, and cover design was performed by Black Dawn Graphics, which has provided services to KoPubCo since 1983.

Dr. K's Sure-Fire Instant Weight-Loss Secrets

Index

Eat.............16, 20, 24, 28, 32, 36, 40, 44, 48, 52, 56, ...60, 64, 68, 72, 76, 80, 84, 88, 92, 96

Exercise ....17, 21, 25, 29, 33, 37, 41, 45, 49, 53, 57, ...61, 65, 69, 73, 77, 81, 85, 89, 93, 97

Insanely...61

Less................16, 20, 24, 28, 32, 36, 40, 44, 48, 52, ...56, 64, 68, 72, 76, 80, 84, 88, 92, 96

More............17, 21, 25, 29, 33, 37, 41, 45, 49, 53, 57, ...60, 61, 65, 69, 73, 77, 81, 85, 89, 93, 97

Coming Soon from KoPubCo

What Color Is Your Stool?

by Victor Koman, MBA

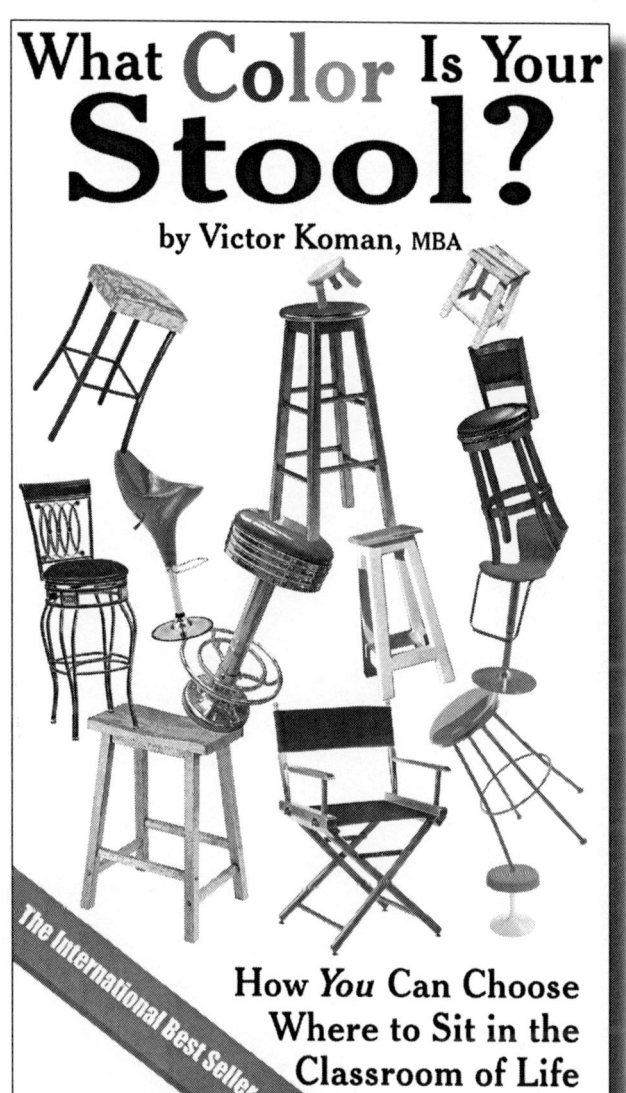

The International Best Seller

How *You* Can Choose Where to Sit in the Classroom of Life